THE POWER OF NATURAL HEALING

MORTAGY RASHED
HEALTH SPECIALIST

Introduction

Natural healing is the practice of using natural remedies and techniques to support the body's natural healing process. From herbal remedies to meditation and acupuncture, there are many natural methods available to help restore and maintain health. In this ebook, we will explore the power of natural healing and how it can be used to support overall health and well-being.

Have you ever wondered about the healing power of nature? From the fresh air, we breathe to the foods we eat, nature has a remarkable ability to restore and maintain our health and well-being. In a world filled with synthetic remedies and pharmaceuticals, it's easy to forget that the natural world has provided us with powerful healing tools for centuries. This ebook is your guide to unlocking the power of natural healing and harnessing the full potential of nature to support your health and vitality. Whether you're dealing with a specific health issue or simply looking to live a healthier, more vibrant life, the techniques and remedies in this ebook will help you tap into the healing power of nature and achieve a greater sense of well-being.

With a deep understanding of the science and history of natural healing, this ebook will help you explore the many benefits of natural remedies and techniques. From herbal remedies to meditation, we will dive into the different types of natural healing methods and their specific benefits. We will also provide practical guidance on how to create a natural healing plan that works for you and incorporate natural healing methods into your daily routine.

In addition to discussing how natural healing can help with specific health issues, we will also explore how it can be used to support a healthy lifestyle. This includes everything from making healthy food choices to developing a healthy mindset and maintaining a healthy environment.

With this comprehensive guide to natural healing, you will discover the many ways that nature can help you achieve optimal health and well-being. So whether you're a a seasoned practitioner of natural healing or just starting to explore this powerful approach, this ebook is the perfect resource for anyone looking to unlock the healing power of nature and live a healthier, more vibrant life.

In today's fast-paced and stress-filled world, natural healing has become increasingly popular as people look for alternative ways to support their health and well-being. This ebook is designed to provide a comprehensive overview of natural healing, including its history, science, benefits, and various techniques.

Through exploring the different types of natural healing methods, you will learn how to use the power of nature to support your body's natural healing process. Whether you're looking to alleviate chronic pain, reduce stress and anxiety, or simply maintain optimally health, the techniques and remedies in this ebook will provide you with a powerful toolkit for supporting your health and vitality.

By incorporating natural healing into your daily routine, you can take control of your health and well-being and reduce your reliance on synthetic remedies and pharmaceuticals. With a focus on self-care and developing healthy habits, this ebook will guide you on your journey to better health and vitality.

So if you're ready to tap into the power of nature and unlock the healing potential that lies within, this ebook is the perfect resource for you. With its practical guidance and comprehensive approach to natural healing, you will be empowered to take charge of your health and live a healthier, more vibrant life.

Chapter 1: Understanding Natural Healing

Understanding natural healing begins with recognizing that the body has an innate ability to heal itself. Natural healing is a holistic approach that aims to support the body's natural healing process by addressing the underlying causes of illness and disease.

To understand natural healing, it is important to learn about the different types of natural healing methods, such as herbal remedies, acupuncture, massage therapy, meditation, and yoga. Each method works in different ways to support the body's natural healing process and promote overall health and well-being.

It is also important to understand the benefits of natural healing, which include improved physical and mental health, increased energy and vitality, and reduced stress and anxiety. Natural healing can also help prevent illness and disease by supporting the immune system and improving overall health.

Developing a natural healing plan that works for you is also an important part of understanding natural healing. This includes incorporating healthy habits into your daily routine, such as eating a healthy diet, getting regular exercise, practicing self-care, and incorporating natural healing methods into your daily routine.

Finally, it is important to recognize that natural healing is a journey, and it may take time to see the full benefits of these methods. It is important to be patient and persistent in your approach and to seek guidance and support from qualified practitioners as needed.

By developing an understanding of natural healing and incorporating these methods into your daily routine, you can tap into the healing power of nature and support your body's natural healing process. With time and practice, you can achieve optimal health and well-being, and live a healthier, more vibrant life.

Natural healing is a multidisciplinary field that draws on a wide range of traditional and modern practices. It recognizes the interconnectedness of the body, mind, and spirit and emphasizes the importance of addressing all aspects of a person's well-being. This holistic approach aims to not only alleviate specific health issues but also to promote overall health and vitality.

Understanding natural healing also involves understanding the role of natural remedies in supporting the body's natural healing process. This includes the use of herbs, vitamins, minerals, and other natural substances to support the body's natural healing mechanisms. Natural remedies can be used to address a wide range of health issues, from common colds and flu to chronic conditions like arthritis, diabetes, and heart disease.

In addition to natural remedies, natural healing also involves lifestyle changes and mind-body practices. These practices, such as meditation, yoga, and tai chi, can help reduce stress and anxiety, promote relaxation, and improve overall health and well-being.

To fully understand natural healing, it is important to recognize that it is not a one-size-fits-all approach. Each person's body is unique and responds differently to different treatments. It is important to work with a qualified practitioner to develop a personalized natural healing plan that takes into account your individual needs and health concerns.

Chapter 2: Benefits of Natural Healing

Natural healing has a wide range of benefits for both the body and the mind. Here are some unique benefits of natural healing:

1. Natural remedies are gentle and safe: Natural remedies, such as herbs and essential oils, are gentle and safe and have few side effects when used appropriately. This makes them a great alternative to pharmaceuticals that can often have harmful side effects.
2. Natural healing supports the body's natural healing process: Natural healing methods, such as acupuncture and massage therapy, work to support the body's natural healing mechanisms. By addressing the root causes of illness and disease, natural healing can promote lasting health and vitality.
3. Natural healing is non-invasive: Many natural healing methods, such as meditation and yoga, are non-invasive and do not require surgery or other invasive procedures. This makes them a great option for those who want to avoid the risks and discomfort associated with more invasive treatments.
4. Natural healing is sustainable: Natural healing methods focus on developing healthy habits and making sustainable lifestyle changes. By incorporating these practices into your daily routine, you can promote long-term health and well-being.
5. Natural healing is cost-effective: Natural remedies and lifestyle changes are often more cost-effective than pharmaceuticals and medical procedures. This makes natural healing an accessible option for those on a budget or without access to traditional medical care.

In addition to the unique benefits listed above, natural healing has a wide range of additional benefits for the body and the mind. Here are a few more benefits of natural healing to consider:

1. Natural healing can improve immune function: Many natural remedies, such as echinacea and elderberry, are known for their immune-boosting properties. By incorporating these remedies into your routine, you can support your body's natural defenses and reduce your risk of illness and infection.

2. Natural healing can reduce stress and anxiety: Mind-body practices, such as meditation and yoga, can be powerful tools for reducing stress and anxiety. By learning to manage stress in a healthy way, you can promote overall well-being and reduce your risk of stress-related illness.

3. Natural healing can improve sleep: Many natural remedies and lifestyle changes, such as herbal teas and a regular sleep schedule, can improve sleep quality and duration. By getting enough sleep, you can promote overall health and vitality and reduce your risk of chronic illness.

4. Natural healing can promote healthy digestion: Many natural remedies, such as ginger and peppermint, are known for their digestive benefits. By incorporating these remedies into your routine, you can support healthy digestion and reduce your risk of digestive issues like bloating and constipation.

5. Natural healing can support mental health: In addition to reducing stress and anxiety, natural healing practices like aromatherapy and herbal remedies can support mental health and promote feelings of calm and relaxation.

Chapter 3: Natural Healing Techniques

Natural healing techniques encompass a wide range of traditional and modern practices that aim to support the body's natural healing mechanisms. Here are some unique natural healing techniques to consider:

1. Acupuncture: Acupuncture is a traditional Chinese medicine technique that involves inserting thin needles into specific points on the body. This practice is believed to balance the body's energy flow and promote healing.
2. Herbal remedies: Herbal remedies are plant-based products, such as teas and tinctures, that are used to support the body's natural healing mechanisms. Different herbs have different properties and can be used to address a wide range of health issues.
3. Massage therapy: Massage therapy involves manipulating the body's soft tissues to promote relaxation, reduce pain, and improve circulation. This practice can be helpful for a wide range of conditions, from chronic pain to anxiety and depression.
4. Mind-body practices: Mind-body practices, such as meditation, yoga, and tai chi, are techniques that aim to promote relaxation, reduce stress, and improve overall well-being. These practices can help improve physical and mental health and reduce the risk of chronic illness.
5. Aromatherapy: Aromatherapy involves using essential oils, which are derived from plants, to promote relaxation and improve overall well-being. Different oils

have different properties and can be used to address a wide range of health issues.

6. Nutrition and dietary changes: Nutrition and dietary changes can be used to support overall health and promote healing. By focusing on a diet rich in whole, nutrient-dense foods, you can support your body's natural healing mechanisms and reduce your risk of chronic illness.

In addition to the natural healing techniques mentioned above, there are a few more unique techniques to consider:

1. Hydrotherapy: Hydrotherapy is the use of water in the treatment of disease and the promotion of health. This technique involves the use of water in different forms, such as hot or cold compresses, steam baths, or hydro-massage, to promote relaxation, reduce pain, and improve circulation.
2. Chiropractic care: Chiropractic care is a holistic healthcare approach that focuses on the musculoskeletal and nervous systems. This technique involves the use of manual adjustments to the spine and other parts of the body to reduce pain, improve the range of motion, and promote healing.
3. Light therapy: Light therapy, also known as phototherapy, is a non-invasive technique that involves exposure to specific wavelengths of light to promote healing. This technique can be used to treat a range of conditions, such as seasonal affective disorder, sleep disorders, and skin conditions.
4. Energy healing: Energy healing is a practice that involves working with the body's energy fields to promote healing. This technique includes practices like Reiki, Qigong, and healing touch.

5. Movement therapies: Movement therapies, such as dance therapy and Pilates, can be used to promote physical and mental health. These practices focus on movement and breathing to improve strength, flexibility, and overall well-being.

Chapter 4: Creating a Natural Healing Plan

Creating a natural healing plan can help you address your specific health needs and promote lasting wellness. Here are the key steps to consider when creating your own natural healing plan:

1. Assess your health needs: The first step in creating a natural healing plan is to assess your current health needs. Consider your health goals, any health issues you are currently experiencing, and any lifestyle factors that may be contributing to your health concerns.
2. Research natural healing techniques: Once you have a clear understanding of your health needs, research natural healing techniques that can help address your specific issues. Consider different techniques, such as acupuncture, massage therapy, and herbal remedies, and identify the ones that resonate with you.
3. Find qualified practitioners: When working with natural healing techniques, it is important to work with qualified practitioners who can guide you through the process. Research practitioners in your area and choose those who are licensed or certified in their field.
4. Develop a personalized plan: Work with your chosen practitioners to develop a personalized natural healing plan. This plan may include a combination of

different techniques, such as acupuncture, massage therapy, and herbal remedies, as well as dietary and lifestyle changes.

5. Implement your plan: Once you have developed your natural healing plan, it is time to implement it. This may involve scheduling regular appointments with your practitioners, making changes to your diet and lifestyle, and incorporating natural healing techniques into your daily routine.

6. Monitor your progress: As you implement your natural healing plan, monitor your progress and make adjustments as needed. This may involve tracking changes in your symptoms or overall health, and communicating regularly with your practitioners.

When creating a natural healing plan, it is important to keep in mind that natural healing techniques work best as part of a holistic approach to health. This means that in addition to natural healing techniques, it is important to make healthy lifestyle choices that support your overall well-being.

Here are some lifestyle changes that can support your natural healing plan:

1. Eat a healthy diet: Eating a healthy, nutrient-dense diet can provide your body with the building blocks it needs to heal and regenerate. Incorporate plenty of fresh fruits and vegetables, whole grains, lean protein sources, and healthy fats into your diet.

2. Get enough sleep: Getting enough sleep is essential for overall health and well-being. Aim for 7-8 hours of sleep per night, and establish a regular sleep routine to promote restful sleep.

3. Exercise regularly: Regular exercise can help reduce stress, improve circulation, and support overall health. Choose a form of exercise that you enjoy, and aim for at least 30 minutes of moderate-intensity exercise most days of the week.

4. Manage stress: Chronic stress can contribute to a range of health issues, so it is important to manage stress as part of your natural healing plan. Incorporate stress-reducing techniques, such as meditation, yoga, or deep breathing, into your daily routine.

5. Avoid toxins: Toxins in the environment, such as pollutants and chemicals, can contribute to health issues. To support your natural healing plan, avoid exposure to toxins as much as possible. Choose organic foods, use natural cleaning products, and avoid smoking and exposure to secondhand smoke.

By incorporating these lifestyle changes into your natural healing plan, you can support your body's natural healing mechanisms and promote lasting health and well-being. Remember, natural healing is a holistic approach to health that involves addressing the root causes of health issues, rather than just treating symptoms. With a comprehensive natural healing plan and a commitment to healthy lifestyle choices, you can achieve optimal health and vitality.

Chapter 5: Natural Healing for Common Health Issues

Natural healing techniques can be effective for a wide range of common health issues. Here are some examples of natural healing techniques that may be helpful for common health issues:

1. Headaches: Acupuncture, massage therapy, and aromatherapy can be effective in treating headaches. Certain herbs, such as feverfew and butterbur, may also be helpful.
2. Stress and anxiety: Mind-body techniques, such as meditation and yoga, can be helpful in reducing stress and anxiety. Herbal remedies, such as passionflower and valerian, may also be beneficial.
3. Digestive issues: Herbal remedies, such as peppermint and ginger, can be helpful for digestive issues, such as bloating and indigestion. Probiotics and dietary changes, such as avoiding trigger foods and eating a high-fiber diet, may also be beneficial.
4. Insomnia: Relaxation techniques, such as deep breathing and guided imagery, can be helpful in promoting restful sleep. Herbal remedies, such as chamomile and lavender, may also be beneficial.

5. Joint pain: Acupuncture, massage therapy, and chiropractic care can be effective in treating joint pain. Certain supplements, such as glucosamine and chondroitin, may also be helpful.

6. Allergies: Herbal remedies, such as stinging nettle and butterbur, can be helpful in reducing allergy symptoms. Avoiding trigger foods and reducing exposure to allergens can also be beneficial.

7. Skin issues: Topical herbal remedies, such as aloe vera and tea tree oil, can be helpful for treating skin issues, such as acne and eczema. Dietary changes, such as avoiding trigger foods and eating a nutrient-dense diet, may also be beneficial.

In addition to the natural healing techniques mentioned above, there are many other natural remedies that may be helpful for specific health issues. Some additional examples include:

1. Cold and flu: Herbal remedies, such as echinacea and elderberry, can be helpful for boosting the immune system and reducing the severity and duration of cold and flu symptoms. Honey and lemon tea can also be helpful for soothing sore throats and coughs.

2. Menstrual cramps: Herbal remedies, such as ginger and turmeric, can be helpful in reducing menstrual cramps. Heat therapy, such as using a hot water bottle, can also be beneficial.

3. High blood pressure: Dietary changes, such as reducing salt intake and eating a diet rich in fruits and vegetables, can be helpful for reducing high blood pressure. Mind-body techniques, such as meditation and deep breathing, can also be beneficial.

4. Depression: Mind-body techniques, such as mindfulness meditation and yoga, can be helpful in reducing symptoms of depression. Herbal remedies, such as St. John's wort and ashwagandha, may also be beneficial.

5. Urinary tract infections: Herbal remedies, such as cranberry and uva ursi, can be helpful for reducing the symptoms of urinary tract infections. Drinking plenty of water and avoiding trigger foods, such as spicy or acidic foods, can also be beneficial.

It is important to keep in mind that natural healing techniques are not a substitute for medical treatment. If you are experiencing a health issue, it is important to seek medical advice and work with qualified practitioners who can guide you through the healing process. However, natural healing techniques can be a complementary approach to conventional medical treatment and can help support your body's natural healing mechanisms. By incorporating natural healing techniques into your overall health plan, you can promote optimal health and well-being.

When using natural remedies for common health issues, it is important to keep in mind that everyone's body is different and may respond differently to different remedies. It is also important to work with qualified practitioners who can guide you through the healing process and monitor your progress. With the guidance of qualified practitioners and a commitment to healthy lifestyle choices, natural healing techniques can be a powerful tool for promoting optimal health and well-being.

Chapter 6: Natural Healing for a Healthy Lifestyle

Natural healing can be an effective way to support a healthy lifestyle. Here are some ways that you can incorporate natural healing techniques into your daily life to promote optimal health and well-being:

1. Mind-body techniques: Mind-body techniques, such as meditation, deep breathing, and yoga, can be helpful for reducing stress, improving sleep, and promoting overall well-being. Incorporating these techniques into your daily routine can help you feel more grounded and centered, and can help you manage the stress of daily life.

2. Nutrient-dense diet: Eating a nutrient-dense diet that is rich in fruits, vegetables, whole grains, and lean protein can provide your body with the nutrients it needs to function at its best. Incorporating natural remedies, such as herbs and spices, into your meals can also provide additional health benefits.

3. Physical activity: Regular physical activity is important for maintaining a healthy weight, reducing the risk of chronic diseases, and promoting overall well-being. Activities such as walking, biking, or swimming can be an effective way to incorporate movement into your daily routine.

4. Sleep hygiene: Getting adequate, restful sleep is crucial for overall health and well-being. Establishing a regular sleep schedule, creating a relaxing bedtime routine, and creating a comfortable sleep environment can help you get the restful sleep your body needs.

5. Mindful self-care: Incorporating self-care practices, such as taking a relaxing bath, practicing mindfulness, or spending time in nature, can be an effective way to reduce stress and promote overall well-being.

Incorporating natural healing techniques into your daily life can be an effective way to support a healthy lifestyle. By making small, sustainable changes to your daily routine, you can support your body's natural healing mechanisms and promote optimal health and well-being. Remember, it is important to work with qualified practitioners and seek medical advice when necessary to ensure that you are taking the best possible care of your body and mind.

Natural healing is not just about treating specific health issues, but it is also about promoting a holistic approach to health and well-being. When we focus on natural healing for a healthy lifestyle, we are prioritizing our overall health and well-being, rather than just treating specific symptoms.

In addition to the techniques mentioned above, there are many other natural healing techniques that can be beneficial for promoting a healthy lifestyle. For example:

1. Acupuncture: Acupuncture is a traditional Chinese medicine technique that involves inserting thin needles into specific points on the body to stimulate the body's natural healing processes. Acupuncture can be helpful for a range of health issues, including pain, stress, and digestive issues.

2. Aromatherapy: Aromatherapy involves using essential oils to promote physical and emotional well-being. Different essential oils have different properties and can be used for a range of health issues, from promoting relaxation to boosting energy.

3. Massage therapy: Massage therapy involves using hands-on techniques to promote relaxation, reduce muscle tension, and improve circulation. Massage therapy can be helpful for reducing stress, promoting relaxation, and reducing muscle tension and pain.

4. Herbal medicine: Herbal medicine involves using plant-based remedies to promote health and well-being. Different herbs have different properties and can be used for a range of health issues, from promoting relaxation to boosting energy.

By incorporating these natural healing techniques into our daily lives, we can support our bodies natural healing processes and promote optimal health and well-being. As with any health-related practice, it is important to work with qualified practitioners and seek medical advice when necessary to ensure that we are taking the best possible care of our bodies and minds. With a commitment to natural healing, we can support our bodies and minds in achieving optimal health and well-being.

Conclusion

Natural healing is not just a trend or a fad, it is a way of life that has been practiced for thousands of years. It is based on the idea that the body has the innate ability to heal itself when given the right conditions, and that we can support this natural healing process by using natural remedies and techniques.

Natural healing is a holistic approach to health and well-being that takes into account the physical, emotional, and spiritual aspects of our being. By treating the whole person, rather than just specific symptoms or health issues, natural healing can help us to achieve optimal health and well-being.

Natural healing techniques can be used to complement conventional medical treatments, or they can be used on their own to prevent and treat a wide range of health issues. They can be used to support the body's natural healing processes and promote optimal health and well-being, and they can be adapted to suit individual needs and preferences.

In a world that is becoming increasingly complex and stressful, natural healing offers a simple and effective way to support our health and well-being. By incorporating natural healing techniques into our daily lives, we can promote a healthy lifestyle, reduce stress, boost energy, and support the body's natural healing mechanisms.

Natural healing is a powerful approach to promoting health and well-being that has been practiced for thousands of years. By using natural remedies and techniques, we can support the body's natural healing processes and promote optimal health and well-being. With a commitment to natural healing, we can create a healthier and happier life for ourselves and those around us.